RICHARD A. LANHAM

UNIVERSITY OF CALIFORNIA, LOS ANGELES

The

Revising Prose

Self-Teaching Exercise Book

MACMILLAN PUBLISHING COMPANY
NEW YORK
COLLIER MACMILLAN PUBLISHERS
LONDON

Macmillan Publishing Company
866 Third Avenue, New York, New York 10022

Collier Macmillan Canada, Inc.

Printing: 2 3 4 5 6 7   Year: 9 0 1 2 3

ISBN 0-02-367490-3

CONTENTS

I. EXERCISES

II. COMMENTS AND REVISIONS

HOW TO USE THIS BOOK

This exercise book has two parts. The first, a series of exercises, allows you to solve for yourself prose-revision problems like those discussed in **Revising Prose.** The second, comments and suggested revisions for each exercise, allows you to compare your solutions with mine. I don't offer my revisions as the "right" ones, but only as starting-points for further discussion and revision. If you accept my revisions as the last word, you'll learn much less than you might. If you read my revisions before you do your own, obviously you'll learn nothing at all.

The exercises are not arranged in order of difficulty or by stylistic attribute. They are simply a series of case-studies in academic prose style, all taken from real life, and almost all in need of serious revision. I have not designed them to be used with the book in any particular way; use them however seems best to you. If I were doing it, I would work through them all in conjunction with the first three chapters of the book, and then review them, and my revisions, more reflectively after completing the concluding chapters.

I reprint the Paramedic Method here. As I say in the book, it works only if you use it rather than gingerly dance around it .

As I also say in the book, the Paramedic Method is *paramedicine*, not *medicine;* not a complete theory of prose style but a specific solution for a specific problem - the use of The Official Style in many places where it does not fit. Incurable English teacher that I am, I cherish a fond hope that some readers of this book will get interested in prose analysis in its full range, and want to move from particular case to general theory. If you would like to study the larger picture of which these exercises form a detail, I've written **Analyzing Prose**, also available from Macmillan, to give you a start. **Analyzing Prose** moves the whole affair from *exercise* to *play*, where it really belongs.

THE PARAMEDIC METHOD

1. Circle the prepositions.
2. Circle the "is" forms.
3. Ask "Who is kicking Who?"
4. Put this "kicking" action in a simple (not compound) active verb.
5. Start fast - no mindless introductions.
6. Write out each sentence on a blank sheet of paper and mark off its basic rhythmic units with a "/".
7. Read the passage aloud with emphasis and feeling.
8. Mark off sentence lengths in the passage with a "/".

UNDERGRADUATE PROSE
Sentence Revision

1.   He sees literature's primary function as a manifestation of the realm of imagination.

_____

_____

_____

2.   He is continually obsessed with the longing of death and at times is fascinated with death's peculiar nature.

_____

_____

_____

3.   For the most part, my relationship with my Mentees has been one of friendship.

_____

_____

_____

4.   There is one further comment of Berkeley's, on another topic, which is also supportive of the above premises.

_____

_____

_____

5.   The differences in the presentation and rehearsal times may also have had some effect on the results.

_____

_____

_____

6.   Attempts to explain the Olds-Milner phenomenon have been numerous.

_____

_____

_____

7.   One of the most important indicators of the sensorimotor period is the gradual development of object permanence.

_____

_____

_____

8.   During the late fifties and early sixties, a phenomenon is taking place in the family for the first time.

_____

_____

_____

9.   The manner in which behavior first shown in a conflict situation may become fixed so that it persists after the conflict has passed is then discussed.

_____

_____

_____

10.   Before 1750 A.D. the world was characterized by the lack of any urbanization.

_____

_____

_____

11.   A political philosophy that was evident in all stable preindustrial cities was Capitalism.

_____

_____

_____

12. The excerpt is an increment in the process of informing the reader regarding the characters by permitting the reader to infer from events rather than accept a description.

_____

_____

_____

_____

13.   By individuals internalizing and conforming to rules which are enforced by authority, a harmonious social structure is maintained.

_____

_____

_____

14.   This paper presents an analysis of variations in the relative abundances of common primary elements arising from differences in the lifetime of the progenitor stars.

_____

_____

_____

15.   It must suffice to say that the traditional values, in which the goal is prosperity and stability, eudaimonia, and the agathos, the man whose characteristics are commended by arete, is the prosperous, brave and successful man, are still dominant.

_____

_____

_____

_____

16.   The more ingenious opponents of preferential treatment are currently arguing that the preferential awarding of grades in university courses, such as Philosophy 4, can be justified for all the same reasons relied upon to justify preferential treatment in hiring and admissions.

_____

_____

_____

17. In the case of finding a set of premises that are beyond our limited means of verification, all we can say about the belief we originally set out to judge is that it is as certain, and no more certain, as these fundamental premises are.

---

18. Due to the many false connotations radiated throughout Cinderella, this fairy tale may prove to be a influence on children, and harmful to them during the course of their lives.

---

19. Along these lines, it is essential to note that black women, as a whole, tend to start work earlier, as is exemplified by Anne Moody who began doing domestic work for a white woman at about the age of 10 years for 75 cents a week plus milk, work longer and make less money.

---

20. Thirdly, elimination of all the professionals and intellectuals took place by arresting them.

_____

_____

_____

21. The following experiments are reconstructions of those two significant discoveries.

_____

_____

_____

22. What I hope to accomplish in this report is threefold.

_____

_____

23. The aim of this paper is to contrast Piaget's object permanence theory, which states that infants initially rely on an action memory schema to retrieve a hidden object and then gradually develop object permanence as new schemas are incorporated, to that of Cummings and Bjork (1980).

_____

_____

_____

_____

_____

24. Since I have no plans to write a book about the Weather Service, I will try to be brief, but concise in the ensuing pages.

_____

_____

_____

25.   One suggestion concerning the relationships between the syndrome of Early Infantile Autism and hemispheric specialization was proposed by Tanguay (1972).

_____

_____

_____

Paragraph Revision

1.   Through my educational experiences I have come to the conclusion that school and college specifically is for learning and expanding one's knowledge in many areas, but also for meeting and coming into contact with different cultures and people. College should not just be a place where one learns the mechanical aspects of education, but also should be an experience which helps one to grow in social and mental awareness of the world in order to survive and have a successful career in one's lifetime.

To limit a college education to complete and total existence in a classroom is a dangerous and unhealthy aspect to conceive of happening, because People will be who one must get along with in order to live happily on the job, in the home and out on the streets. Social awareness must also be a part of the educational system. College at the present time is doing an excellent job with keeping students active and informed.

_____

_____

_____

_____

_____

_____

_____

_____

_____

_____

_____

_____

2.　　The procedure for transferring the magnetometer data from the cassette data tapes to the IBM 3033 has been through a number of generations. The end result however is still a disk data file at the Campus Computing System. I have written a number of data manipulation programs to modify the data based on this specific data file.

The first block of such programs transforms the above mentioned data file into a standard data form called the Block Data Set (BDS). The second block of manipulatory programs use the BDS input and then give varying types of output.

---

3.   Ulrich von Lichtenstein achieved a strange mixture of tradition and innovation, fact and fantasy, truth and fiction, artistic virtuosity and dilettantish ineptness in his <u>Service of Ladies</u> completed in 1255. Long a controversial source for information about chivalry and the facts behind the conventions of medieval German love lyrics, despite early objections that this work, commonly regarded as the first German vernacular autobiography, was too indebted to literary models to provide reliable information on cultural history, this conglomeration of an extended narration on the education of a knight of love interspersed with and highlighted by fabliau-like comic episodes, amorous letters and booklets, and some fifty-eight songs, predominantly dealing with questions of love, has attracted a flood of scholarly attention in the past two decades.

_____

_____

_____

_____

_____

_____

_____

_____

_____

_____

_____

_____

_____

_____

_____

4.   Open the fiberglass pit by removing the attachment bolts and carefully lift off the top so as to keep from dropping dirt into the pit. This exposes the top of the instrumentation rack on which the system controller and the magnetometer rest. Using the free black and orange lead connect the display battery (black to negative first). With the battery connected watch the display for three consecutive field readings noting the second on which the battery light turns on and the field value. The three values should be consistent with 10y. The absolute value should be around 50,000y. The consistency is by far the more important of the two because occasionally elements of the display fail making the numbers appear very different.

_____

_____

_____

_____

_____

_____

_____

_____

_____

_____

_____

_____

_____

5. Although Professor Radcliffe-Brown's definition of political organization is to some extent correct, it is both inadequate and inaccurate, especially in its qualifications of the nebulous tenet; political organization is the component of social order, which serves to both stabilize and propagate the social order. To say that political organization is the force that unifies society is to say very little, indeed. The implication that this cohesion is efficacious only within a demarcated boundary under the auspices of a codified instrument of judicious authority is preposterous, when viewed in terms of societies whose social awareness is little more complex than the pectic bond between pack animals.

_____

_____

_____

_____

_____

_____

_____

_____

_____

_____

_____

_____

_____

_____

_____

GRADUATE PROSE

1.   A perfect example of the resultant polluted fragmentation of the Russian intelligentsia may be seen in the characters of Dostoevsky's <u>The Idiot</u>, who have a desperate awareness of the uncertain ground of their actions that causes them to hurl themselves towards a decisive event - revolution, crime, suicide, libertinism, religious extremism - in the hope that the external situation thus created will deprive them of choice and impose unity on their personalities.

_____

_____

_____

_____

_____

_____

_____

_____

_____

2.   As a life-bringer and a death-dealer the old man contains his own opposites, and the hero's destruction of the dualistic greybeard provides a metaphor for the psychological process of incorporating the shadow, or dark side of the personality into the self for the purpose of achieving wholeness. The archetype of the Self represents the fusion of the various components of the psyche into a comprehensive entity, and this paradoxical union of opposites prefigures the phenomenon of rebirth and transfiguration.

_____

_____

_____

_____

_____

_____

_____

_____

_____

3.   Behavior, words and body movements are gestures that evoke similar, identical and unique responses or reactions to the individual or community initiating the gesture. Paradoxically, gestures which create immediate perceptions, may direct or misdirect the person or community trying to interpret the motivation or meaning behind those gestures.

_____

_____

_____

_____

_____

_____

_____

4.   At this stage of the development of the spirit archetype, furthermore, the internalized Spirit would "miraculously" intervene to save the child from death, in spite of the unremitting perilousness of his adventures.

_____

_____

_____

_____

5.   Sex and violence: the two pursuits which express man's strongest physical urges. Every age must cope with them, must devise systems that allow release yet preserve a modicum of control. For the Elizabethans that control almost evaporated. The medieval church had ritualized sex and violence, defined their role in the cosmos. Expanding beyond these religious strictures, the Renaissance intellect faced emotional chaos. Therefore, a cultural preoccupation with these impulses evolved, which only our own age, emerging from the repressive safeguards of Puritanism and Victorianism, can match.

_____

_____

_____

_____

_____

_____

_____

_____

_____

Original and Revision Studies

Passages 6-10 come from graduate papers submitted to me at UCLA and subsequently revised in office-hour visits. Try your hand at revision and then look at the revisions done by the students themselves. What is gained or lost in revision? (Or reverse the process; start with the revision and expand it back into the original version by reversing the Paramedic Method.) The papers all come from an English department, since that is where I teach, but the principles used in revising apply across the curriculum.

6. Original

Yeats's intense fear of skepticism is one of the dominant forces behind his poetry. Born into a world "in which each element is separated from others," a world "that is now but a bundle of garments," Yeats sets out to create a poetry of "complete affirmation" and "unity between man, nature, and the supernatural." Through his romantic longing for the reconciliation of opposites, his compulsion to create an autonomous, comprehensive system of philosophy, his faith in the nobility of tradition and his effort to recover and celebrate it in his poetry, Yeats combats, both internally and externally, the powerful forces of contemporary nihilism. "Profound philosophy must come from terror," wrote Yeats in 1936. At the source of Yeats's poetry and philosophy lies the profoundest fear of existential nausea.

Revision

Yeats's fear of skepticism dominates his poetry. Through a philosophic system which reconciles opposites and celebrates the nobility of tradition Yeats combats contemporary nihilism. "Profound philosophy must come from terror," he wrote in 1936. Yeats's poetry and philosophy springs from his fear of existential nausea.

7. Original

The critical furor which after fifty years still surrounds <u>Ulysses</u> has one of its chief origins in Joyce's fusion of two very different modes of artistic representation, symbolism and realism. Yet, even momentarily putting aside the symbolic elements of <u>Ulysses</u>, we find more problems in examining the level of literal action than we usually encounter in a novel - and not only because the narrative is occasionally obscured or confused by the narrator's intrusions. Joyce greatly extrapolated the novel's historical tendency to de-emphasize plot in favor of character; thus he circumscribes his plot to the events of a single day and also employs narrative methods which emphasize internal activity over external. <u>Ulysses</u> has the scope of a <u>Bildungsroman</u>, but we receive the histories of the characters piecemeal and unordered. Moreover, though access to the characters' thoughts enables us to infer their present situations and to reconstruct their pasts, it does so only to the extent that their thoughts actually match reality. Joyce's is a subjective or psychological realism. It is within the context of the psychological realism that I wish to examine Leopold Bloom.

Revision

The critical furor still surrounding <u>Ulysses</u> stems chiefly from Joyce's fusing of symbolism and realism. And, surprisingly, the realism causes more problems than the symbolism. The allusions don't confuse us much. But Joyce greatly exaggerates the novel's historical tendency to emphasize character over plot. He narrows his story to a single day and narrates more thoughts than acts. <u>Ulysses</u> reads like an exploded <u>Bildungsroman.</u> The characters' histories come piecemeal and unordered. Moreover, as we infer their histories from their memories, we must use a fine filter, for their fantasies and fears continually obscure the facts. At the novel's center, most obscured of all, stands Leopold Bloom.

8.   Original

Surprisingly, the central character in <u>Ulysses</u> has been relatively ignored in many critical discussions. William Schutte makes this point in his article, "Leopold Bloom: A Touch of the Artist": " (Bloom) has all too often been shoved firmly, if usually politely, into the background while discussions have raged about the structural patterning and the manifold techniques of the novel, the uses of irony, or the roles of Molly and Stephen." Often Bloom yields in favor of Stephen, for many critics have tended to read <u>Ulysses</u> primarily as a sequel to Stephen's story in <u>A Portrait of the Artist as a Young Man.</u> I disagree with such readings, and I feel that the best single approach to the central meaning of the novel is through Bloom, its central character. I am not concerned in this paper with Bloom in relation to his many avatars, such as Ulysses, Jesus, Buddha, Elijah, Ahaserus, and Moses.   Rather, largely ignoring these correspondences, I am interested in Bloom on a more literal level, in relation to his family, to Stephen, and to Dublin, that is, in his three major roles as husband, father, and citizen. Within these roles, I believe, Bloom changes during the course of his day; even if we argue, as some critics do, that significant character development is impossible within the space of eighteen hours, I think it remains undeniable that our own understanding of Bloom evolves and changes through the course of the novel.   Although a close examination of this process through each chapter is beyond the scope and outside the intention of this paper, I do outline the major movement of the change by isolating what I consider to be the key passages.

Revision

Critics have largely ignored <u>Ulysses'</u> central character. William Schutte makes this point: ". . . (Bloom) has all too often been shoved firmly, if usually politely, into the background while discussions have raged about the structural patterning and the manifold techniques of the novel, the uses of irony, or the roles of Molly and Stephen." Since many critics read <u>Ulysses</u> as a sequel to <u>A Portrait of the Artist as a Young Man,</u>

Bloom often yields to Stephen. I feel, however, that we should approach the novel through Bloom. His many avatars - Ulysses, Jesus, Buddha, and the rest - don't concern me here. I wish to view Bloom more literally, as husband, father, and citizen. Within these roles, Bloom changes during the novel. Even if a character cannot develop significantly in eighteen hours, our understanding of him can. I want to trace this movement and isolate its major stages.

9. Original

Even a cursory reading of the romances indicates Hawthorne's preoccupation with woman and her role in life. In the creation of certain female characters - for example, Priscilla - he reveals his understanding of the prevalent social myths regarding women and their proper function in life; in the creation of certain male characters - for example, Hollingsworth - he also demonstrates his awareness that the disabilities confronting women are closely related to the problem of masculine egotism. Priscilla incorporates in her nature qualities which suit her to be one of the exploited slaves discussed in Mill's The Subjection of Women as well as one of the ethereal queens praised by Ruskin's "Of Queens' Gardens." That neither of these was yet written when The Blithedale Romance was published only indicates that Hawthorne was in the vanguard of awareness on these issues.

Revision

Hawthorne's preoccupation with women shows up everywhere. Female characters like Priscilla prove that he understands the prevalent myths about women, and male characters like Hollingsworth indicate that he recognizes masculine egotism, too. Some of Priscilla's attributes could qualify her as one of the exploited slaves in Mill's The Subjection of Women, but others suggest the ethereal queens in Ruskin's "Of Queens' Gardens." That The Blithedale Romance precedes both works indicates that Hawthorne had a prophetic sensitivity to woman's plight.

10. Original

Raymond Chandler took part in a miniature, fragmented literary episode in the middle of the twentieth century; its writers, in retrospect, performed the considerable feat of making Los Angeles possible for literature. Some of Chandler's famous partners in this effort - Aldous Huxley, Nathaniel West, F. Scott Fitzgerald, Evelyn Waugh - we still read, respect, and admire. Chandler aspired to their ranks and their standards but writers of mystery and detection remained the base camp for his assault upon the literary heights. Just as Los Angeles once seemed lacking as a literary milieu, critics dismissed mystery writing as formulaic, mercenary, ultramontane. Chandler's public achievement is that he redeemed the locale and the genre for serious literary consideration; but his official success obscures, although it is in no way separate from, his private struggle, survival and eventual triumph.

Revision

During the nineteen thirties and 'forties, Los Angeles, source of so many modern images, acquired one for itself. A group of writers, who were not organized and did not plan this result, performed the considerable feat of making Los Angeles possible for literature. Some of these writers - Huxley, West, Fitzgerald, Waugh - we still respect, admire, and read. But we are still discovering others who participated in this fragmented episode in literary history. Although Raymond Chandler remains one of the less well-known, yet equally talented authors, an authoritative biography, Frank MacShane's <u>The Life of Raymond Chandler</u>, and a wide-ranging collection of essays, Miriam Gross' <u>The World of Raymond Chandler</u>, substantially contribute to his reputation and to our knowledge of him.

Mystery writing once seemed as formulaic, mercenary, and ultramontane as did Los Angeles itself. But as these two volumes indicate, Chandler aspired to the ranks and standards of serious fiction. He consciously attempted to make mystery writing both more artistic and more realistic; he wanted to improve its standing among literary critics as well as among its audience, who applied the most demanding standards of all: they read for entertainment and escape. But Chandler also produced, perhaps unintentionally, a body of work which today remains the most vivid, evocative written record of Los Angeles.

PROFESSORIAL PROSE

1.   At the center of any theory of a science of society is an image of man, a conception of him as a particular kind of creature, defined by his powers and liabilities.

_____

_____

_____

2.   Perception is the process of extracting information from stimulation emanating from the objects, places, and events in the world around us.

_____

_____

_____

3.   The notion of a process of abstraction at a perceptual level is not a new one.

_____

_____

4.   An excellent example of the use of the most economical distinctive feature for making a perceptual decision is an experiment by Yonas.

_____

_____

_____

5. If we want to facilitate abstraction of a relation (and we often do in educational situations), we can draw attention to it by enhancing the feature contrast, or by providing uncluttered examples of the invariant property.

_____

_____

_____

_____

6. The concept of role differentiation in any social system may be defined as the structures of distribution of the members of the system among the various positions and activities distinguished in the system, and hence the differential arrangement of the members of the system.

_____

_____

_____

_____

_____

7. We feel that a number of books on reading have failed in what should be an important function, that of providing the psychological and linguistic concepts that will give the student of reading insight into the learning process and what it is that must be learned to be a good reader.

_____

_____

_____

_____

_____

8.   The most eloquent testimony of the flexibility and the durability of the academy as an institution is that offered by Arcadia, the pan-Italian federation of local academies founded in Rome in 1690 by the former members of the salon of Queen Christina of Sweden for the purpose of reforming Italian literature in accordance with the literary models of the High Renaissance.

_____

_____

_____

_____

_____

9.   In this paper, we replace the realistic radiative transfer process by an escape probability method for a slab geometry (of iinfinite area but finite thickness). We make this approximation in order to be able to explore a wide range of parameter space. Modifications would have to be made to the escape probability-optical depth relation for a spherical geometry.

_____

_____

_____

_____

_____

10. An awareness of the role of the recording industry in the dissemination of folk music and musical styles is not new; to date, however, there has been little consideration of the importance of commercial recording in relation to Irish folk music.

_____

_____

_____

_____

11. From this description, it can be seen that a positive incremental voltage applied to a device biased beyond the peak in the velocity-field curve causes a decrease in the terminal current due to the formation of the dipole layer. This is a negative resistance.

_____

_____

_____

_____

12. The lot of the prisoner on the battlefield of the gunpowder age benefited from the generalization of the principle of ransom.

_____

_____

_____

13. What makes episodes of this sort so difficult for the modern reader to visualize, if visualized to believe in, if believed in to understand, is precisely their nakedly face-to-face quality, their offering and delivery of death over distances at which suburbanites swap neighbourly gardening hints, their letting of blood and infliction of pain in circumstances of human congestion we expect to experience only at cocktail parties or tennis tournaments.

_____

_____

_____

_____

_____

_____

_____

14. The same scheme was adopted for the promotion of the study of the church fathers and of the implications of humanism for ecclesiastical reform by the Tridentine enthusiasts in the entourage of the young cardinal Carlo Borromeo during the pontificate of his uncle, Pius IV.

_____

_____

_____

_____

15. On the other hand, the firmness (or rigidity) of some university faculties, including my own, in resisting the awarding of credit for remedial work arises directly out of their sense of vulnerability of the standards for college level work, standards already weakened by diversity, competition, a shocking grade inflation since the mid-1960s, the powerful pressure of the market for enrollments and the call for "relevance." The fact that there are differences on this matter, both of views and of practice, is the best evidence for how soft is the concept of academic standards in higher education, and consequently how vulnerable those standards are to market pressures, especially the pressure to maintain enrollment at all costs.

_____

_____

_____

_____

_____

_____

_____

_____

_____

_____

16. During the year ahead it is my intention to engage a larger number of incumbent faculty in the governance process.

_____

_____

_____

17. The limitations along another dimension of sociobiological explanations of human social activity can be illustrated by considering the Cartesian product of the act/action distinction with the distinction between activities which have a biological origin in an inherited genetic program selected by Darwinian processes, and those which have their origin in the creative cognitive activities of men as conscious social beings.

_____

_____

_____

_____

_____

_____

18. The progress of the discipline of psychoanalysis is expressed perhaps most obviously in its theory of transference and the therapeutic effects of the interpretation of transference.

_____

_____

_____

19. My main reason for writing this book is to reassert the methodological priority of the search for the laws of history in the science of man. There is an urgency associated with this rededication, which grows in direct proportion to the increase in the funding and planning of anthropological research and especially to the role anthropologists have been asked to assume in the planning and carrying out of international development programs. A general theory of history is required if the expansion of disposable research funds is to result in something other than the rapid growth in the amount of trivia being published in the learned journals.

_____

_____

_____

_____

_____

_____

_____

_____

_____

20. Our lives and the world we are part of are uniquely multifaceted and a sense of identity with this pluralism is expressed in musical terms. The fact that there are today so many varied aesthetic attitudes shaping the musical structures and that these approaches to creativity are seemingly disparate is consciously understood and challenged. That as we live side by side and with and among so many attitudes, so music's language is a host that embraces a wide range of possibilities.

_____

_____

_____

_____

_____

_____

UNDERGRADUATE PROSE
Sentence Revision

1. He sees literature's primary function as a manifestation of the realm of imagination.

Comment: You notice the "shun" words first: func**tion**, manifesta**tion**, imagina**tion**. Then the laundry list:

>   **as** a manifestation

>   **of** the realm

>   **of** imagination.

The *shun* words all shunt the potential **action** off into nouns striving to breathe: "function" wants to **act**; "manifestation" wants to **manifest** or **make something plain**; "imagination" wants to **imagine**. All those frustrated incipient actions blur the prose, cloud the central action. And if you are talking of literature's *primary* function, then you can just tell us what that is, without the adjective "primary" at all. Nor do you need to qualify "imagination" with "realm of." You can see here how the vague thinking is constructed by mistakes at the sentence level: too much suppressed and conflicting action; too much qualification ("primary" and "realm of"); and a construction which starts out with "He" as the subject but then spends most of its length talking about another subject - "literature." Amazing how many confusions a 13-word sentence can launch. Here are two revisions. They both illustrate the sentence's final weakness: a vapid banality that borders on tautology. But this weak thinking can be seen, and cured, only by this kind of tedious sentence-level revision. Once you see the problems here, the solution - back for some fresh thinking - emerges of itself.

Revisions:
1. Literature, he thinks, manifests the imagination.
2. He sees literature as manifesting the imagination.

2.   He is continually obsessed with the longing of death and at times is fascinated with death's peculiar nature.

Comment: Perfect for PM revision: He *is* continually obsessed *with* the longing *of* death and *at* times *is* fascinated *with* death's peculiar nature. It should be longing *for* death and not longing *of* death, of course. And what does "death's peculiar nature" mean?

Revision: He continually longs for death and is sometimes fascinated by it.

3. For the most part, my relationship with my Mentees has been one of friendship.

Comment: A perfect instance of ordinary utterance deformed by The Official Style.

Revision: Mostly, I have liked my Mentees.

4. There is one further comment of Berkeley's, on another topic, which is also supportive of the above premises.

Comment: Berkeley is the actor, so let him comment; "is also supportive" means "support," so let him support, too.

Revision: Berkeley, commenting on another topic, supports these premises.

5. The differences in the presentation and rehearsal times may also have had some effect on the results.

Comment: The continual Official Style blurring of simple verbs into compound forms - "had some effect on" for "affect" - bleeds the life out of prose. The rest is a snap. The Lard Factor is only 35%, but the focus improves dramatically.

Revision: Our different presentation and rehearsal times may have affected the results.

6. Attempts to explain the Olds-Milner phenomenon have been numerous.

Comment: You could say: (1) Many scientists have attempted to explain the Olds-Milner phenomenon; or (2) There have been many attempts to explain the Olds-Milner phenomenon; but neither really improves things much. This sentence presents in classic form a sentence which wants to be a subordinate clause, a point which wants to be made on the way to a more important one. So a revision looks like this.

Revision: We might ask why the many attempts to explain the Olds-Milner phenomenon have all failed.

7. One of the most important indicators of the sensorimotor period is the gradual development of object permanence.

Comment: Classic Official Style laundry list:
One

> **of** the most important indicators
>
> **of** the sensorimotor period
>
> **is** the gradual development
>
> **of** object permanence.

Prose like this is not really bad or hard to understand. It is written almost automatically, by the "is plus prepositional phrase" formula. And, in this case, it is not all that easy to fix. Here are some attempts. Are they any better than the original? Do they change its meaning?

Revisions:
1. In the sensorimotor period object permanence gradually develops.
2. The sensorimotor period is indicated most importantly by the gradual development of object permanence.
3. The gradual development of object permanence provides one of the most important indicators of the sensorimotor period.

8. During the late fifties and early sixties, a phenomenon is taking place in the family for the first time.

Comment: All the problems come in the second half: "phenomenon" is vague enough, and then comes the list, is taking place/in the family/for the first time. You have to rephrase entirely.

Revision: During the late 50's and early 60's, something new happens in the family.

9. The manner in which behavior first shown in a conflict situation may become fixed so that it persists after the conflict has passed is then discussed.

Comment: Easy to fix:

The manner in which behavior first shown in a~~~ conflict ~~situation~~ may ~~become fixed so that it~~ persists after ᴧwards ~~the conflict has passed~~ is then discussed.

So two revisions present themselves.

Revisions:
1. How behavior first shown in conflict persists later is then discussed.
2. I then discuss how behavior first shown in conflict persists later.

10. Before 1750 A.D. the world was characterized by the lack of any urbanization.

Comment: Easy to diagram:

lacked

Before 1750 A.D. the world ~~was characterized by~~ ~~the~~ lack ~~of any~~ urbanization.

Revisions:
1. Before 1750 A.D. the world lacked urbanization.
2. Before 1750 A.D. the world was not urbanized.
3. Urbanization occurred only after 1750 A.D.

11. A political philosophy that was evident in all stable preindustrial cities was Capitalism.

Comment: The worst problem here: the "was . . . was" repetition. Next, you have to wonder what "was evident" really means. Existed as a philosophy? Was practiced? Start the sentence off with its natural subject - Capitalism.

Revisions:

1. Capitalism existed in all stable preindustrial citites.

2. Capitalism existed as a political philosophy in all stable preindustrial cities.

3. All stable preindustrial cities knew capitalism as a political philosophy.

12. The excerpt is an increment in the process of informing the reader regarding the characters by permitting the reader to infer from events rather than accept a description.

Comment: A horrendous list:

The excerpt

> **is** an increment

> **in** the process

> **of** informing the reader

> **regarding** the character

> **by** permitting the reader

> **to** infer

> **from** events

This kind of sentence lies awash in quasi-actions:

> The *excerpt* is an *increment* in the *process* of *informing* the reader *regarding* the characters by *permitting* the reader to *infer* from events rather than *accept* a *description.*

So, first, settle on a central action to go with "excerpt" - let's try "permits." All the intervening almost-actions go into the trash. Then, what to do about "accept a description"? It confuses actor and action; who is acting, reader or text? When you think about it - and this is what revising makes you do - "infer" and "accept" are not the opposites the writer thinks they are. Here is the rooted fuzzy thought. A writer can describe events and still ask the reader to infer something from them. You really have to recast the whole sentence.

Revision: In this excerpt, the reader sees the characters in action rather than reading a description of them.

13. By individuals internalizing and conforming to rules which are enforced by authority, a harmonious social structure is maintained.

Comment: Again, the lines of action are blurred. You don't know what action happens first, for a start; and every possible action - internalizing, conforming, enforcing, maintaining - floats at the same level of significance. As so often with The Official Style, you begin at the casting office: you pick a principal actor and action. Then you make some simple equations: "harmonious social structure" = "harmonious society"; "individuals" = "people"; "rules enforced by authority" = "external rules" (we infer that they are external since they are in a contrastive construction with "internal"). Some possible paths out of the wilderness as these equations are progressively put in force.

Revisions:
1. A harmonious society is created by individuals who have internalized external rules.
2. Individuals maintain a harmonious social structure by internalizing external rules.
3. People create a harmonious society by internalizing external rules. (LF. 50%)

14. This paper presents an analysis of variations in the relative abundances of common primary elements arising from differences in the lifetime of the progenitor stars.

Comment: The usual list:

an analysis

of variations

in the relative abundances

of common primary elements arising

from differences

in the lifetime

of the progenitor stars.

Notice how the chain of causality is confused here? No central action is isolated. Instead, a string of verbs and nouns which suggest action of some sort: presents, analysis, variations, abundances, arising, differences, progenitor. You must ask who is doing what to what, Who is kicking Who? The obvious translations present themselves: "presents an analysis of" = "analyze"; "arising from differences in" = "according to." Do you see the transformation that occurs when you concentrate on a single rule - get rid of the prepositions! - and what happens?

Revisions:
1. This paper analyzes how the relative abundance of common primary elements varies with the lifetime of the progenitor stars.
2. This paper analyzes how common primary elements vary in relative abundance with the lifetime of the progenitor stars. (See how this differs from the previous revision? I have put "vary" next to its natural subject, "primary elements.")

15. It must suffice to say that the traditional values, in which the goal is prosperity and stability, eudaimonia, and the agathos, the man whose characteristics are commended by arete, is the prosperous, brave and successful man, are still dominant.

Comment: The main problem, that long apposition floating in mid-sentence, jumps out at you : It must suffice to say that the traditional values, *in which the goal is prosperity and stability, eudaimonia, and the agathos, the man whose characteristics are commended by arete, is the prosperous, brave and successful man,* are still dominant. The apposition floats because "man," unless you know Greek and know that <u>ho agathos</u> means "the good man," has nothing to refer back to. You read it as an absolute quality like the preceding ones - prosperity, stability, and eudaimonia.   Let's begin with the main sentence and leave the appositive until later. "It must suffice to say that," the typical dead-rocket opening, gets cut first.   That uncovers the natural subject, "traditional values," and that in turn uncovers the natural verb, "dominate," or, used without an object, "predominate." The pure stuffing of "in which the goal is" goes up the spout, too.   And the appositive interruption, "the man whose characteristics are commended by arete, is the prosperous, brave and successful man" now stands out as a complete sentence, floating as an appositive in another complete sentence. It turns out to be just a very long-winded way to say "arete."   The final revision, which yields a LF of 72%, shows why it has taken us so long to spell out just how this sentence shoots itself in its own foot.   By no means an extraordinary example of undergraduate prose, it shows how deeply and persistently a writer spellbound by The Official Style can muddle his own processes of thought. The result? An enormous waste of time and energy.

Revision: The traditional values of prosperity, stability, eudaimonia, and arete, still predominate. (LF. 72%)

16. The more ingenious opponents of preferential treatment are currently arguing that the preferential awarding of grades in university courses, such as Philosophy 4, can be justified for all the same reasons relied upon to justify preferential treatment in hiring and admissions.

Comment: The sentence is just too long. A little judicious cutting brings it within bounds.

Revision: The more ingenious opponents of preferential grading argue that it can be justified for the same reasons used to justify preferential hiring and admissions.

17. In the case of finding a set of premises that are beyond our limited means of verification, all we can say about the belief we originally set out to judge is that it is as certain, and no more certain, as these fundamental premises are.

Comment: Let's consider a possible revision and then continue the comment:

> **Revision:** A belief is no more certain than the premises by which we judge it. (LF. 69%)

Does this revision limit the original's meaning? I don't think so. It just focuses its thought much more sharply. Philosophers usually justify their notoriously bad prose by arguing that the intricacies of their thought demand it. Usually, as here, that's applesauce.

18. Due to the many false connotations radiated throughout Cinderella, this fairy tale may prove to be a influence on children, and harmful to them during the course of their lives.

Comment: Mostly pure guff. We don't know what "false connotations" are here but we're stuck with them. The rest is a snap. The revision, as so often, reveals the need for more thinking.

Revision: Cinderella's false connotations may harm children. (LF. 80%)

19. Along these lines, it is essential to note that black women, as a whole, tend to start work earlier, as is exemplified by Anne Moody who began doing domestic work for a white woman at about the age of 10 years for 75 cents a week plus milk, work longer and make less money.

Comment: Let me use different type fonts to suggest what goes with what, and so what is wrong, in this sentence:

Along these lines, it is essential to note that **black women,** as a whole, tend to **start work earlier,** as is exemplified by Anne Moody who began doing domestic work for a white woman at about the age of 10 years for 75 cents a week plus milk, **work longer and make less money.**

Arrivederci the dead-rocket opening and needless later qualifications, and put the example in a separate sentence.

Revision: Black women start work earlier, work longer, and make less money. Anne Moody, for example, began working as a white woman's maid when she was ten years old, for 75 cents a week plus milk.

20. Thirdly, elimination of all the professionals and intellectuals took place by arresting them.

Comment: A classic case of blurring the action between two verbs - eliminate and arrest. Choose one.

Revision:
1. Third, the professionals and intellectuals were arrested.
2. Third, he eliminated the professionals and intellectuals by arresting them all.

21. The following experiments are reconstructions of those two significant discoveries.

Revision: The following experiments reconstruct those two significant discoveries.

22. What I hope to accomplish in this report is threefold.

Revision: This report does three things.

23. The aim of this paper is to contrast Piaget's object permanence theory, which states that infants initially rely on an action memory schema to retrieve a hidden object and then gradually develop object permanence as new schemas are incorporated, to that of Cummings and Bjork (1980).

Comment: A delicatessen-sandwich sentence. Too much filling between the slices of bread.

> The aim of this paper is to contrast Piaget's object permanence theory

> which states that infants initially rely on an action memory schema to retrieve a hidden object and then gradually develop object permanence as new schemas are incorporated,

> to that of Cummings and Bjork (1980).

Solution: Two sentences.

Revision: Piaget's object permanence theory states that infants rely on an action memory schema to retrieve a hidden object and then gradually develop object permanence as new schemas are incorporated. This paper compares Piaget's theory to Cummings and Bjork's (1980).

24. Since I have no plans to write a book about the Weather Service, I will try to be brief, but concise in the ensuing pages.

Comment: Non-funny joke plus a contradictory tautology. "Brief" and "concise" are synonyms but the writer implies by his "but" that they differ in meaning. Solution: bag the joke and be brief about being concise.

Revision: I will be brief.

25. One suggestion concerning the relationships between the syndrome of Early Infantile Autism and hemispheric specialization was proposed by Tanguay (1972).

Revision: Tanguay (1972) suggested that the syndrome of Early Infantile Autism was related to hemispheric specialization in this way: (specify way).

Paragraph Revision

1. Through my educational experiences I have come to the conclusion that school and college specifically is for learning and expanding one's knowledge in many areas, but also for meeting and coming into contact with different cultures and people. College should not just be a place where one learns the mechanical aspects of education, but also should be an experience which helps one to grow in social and mental awareness of the world in order to survive and have a successful career in one's lifetime.

To limit a college education to complete and total existence in a classroom is a dangerous and unhealthy aspect to conceive of happening, because People will be who one must get along with in order to live happily on the job, in the home and out on the streets. Social awareness must also be a part of the educational system. College at the present time is doing an excellent job with keeping students active and informed.

Comment: It is easy to revise this into a sentence or two:

> **Revision:** In college, students should learn not only from books but from their fellow-students; they should grow not only in intellectual maturity but in social awareness as well.

Or some such. But what does such a revision lose? Can you devise a way to preserve the writer's "theme and variations" structure and yet not be so long-winded?

2. The procedure for transferring the magnetometer data from the cassette data tapes to the IBM 3033 has been through a number of generations. The end result however is still a disk data file at the Campus Computing System. I have written a number of data manipulation programs to modify the data based on this specific data file.

The first block of such programs transforms the above mentioned data file into a standard data form called the Block Data Set (BDS). The second block of manipulatory programs use the BDS input and then give varying types of output.

Comment: A few problems (it isn't clear what "based" modifies, "block" needs "uses" not "use," and the first two sentences can be joined) but nothing not easily fixed.

Revision: The procedure for transferring the magnetometer data from the cassette data tapes to the IBM 3033 has been through many generations but still results in a disk data file at the Campus Computing System. I have written several data manipulation programs, based on this specific data file, to modify the data.

The first block of such programs transforms this data file into a standard data form called the Block Data Set (BDS). The second block of manipulatory programs uses the BDS input to produce varying outputs.

3. Ulrich von Lichtenstein achieved a strange mixture of tradition and innovation, fact and fantasy, truth and fiction, artistic virtuosity and dilettantish ineptness in his <u>Service of Ladies</u> completed in 1255. Long a controversial source for information about chivalry and the facts behind the conventions of medieval German love lyrics, despite early objections that this work, commonly regarded as the first German vernacular autobiography, was too indebted to literary models to provide reliable information on cultural history, this conglomeration of an extended narration on the education of a knight of love interspersed with and highlighted by fabliau-like comic episodes, amorous letters and booklets, and some fifty-eight songs, predominantly dealing with questions of love, has attracted a flood of scholarly attention in the past two decades.

Comment: The first sentence needs only a basic inversion to lend it a sense of climax.

> **Revision:** In his <u>Service of Ladies</u>, Ulrich von Lichtenstein achieved a strange mixture of tradition and innovation, fact and fantasy, truth and fiction, artistic virtuosity and dilettantish ineptness.

The second, a hopeless bog of subordination, needs radical surgery. For a start, let's just list the various statements in outline without worrying about their relationship:

1. Long a source for information about chivalry and medieval German love lyrics
2. commonly regarded as the first German vernacular autobiography
3. too indebted to literary models to provide reliable cultural information
4. conglomeration of narrative interspersed with fabliaux, etc.
5. has attracted lots of scholarly attention in last two decades

How might these be sensibly related? Well, we might start with (5) as an introduction. But *what* has attracted a lot of attention? How about (2) next: it is the first German vernacular autobiography. Then (4) follows naturally - a further description of it. Then (1), long a source, etc., but - caution - (3) not a reliable source. The revision proceeds on this basis. But before we revise, reflect for a minute on the magnitude of the error here, the radical failures of thought. If a comparable mistake had been made in a physics lab, it probably would have blown up the apparatus.

Revision: The <u>Service of Ladies</u> has attracted much scholarly attention in the last two decades. An extended narrative interspersed with fabliaux, amorous letters and booklets, and fifty-eight songs, it has long been regarded as the first German vernacular autobiography. Although it tells us much about chivalry and the facts behind courtly love, it is too indebted to literary models to provide wholly-reliable cultural history.

4. Open the fiberglass pit by removing the attachment bolts and carefully lift off the top so as to keep from dropping dirt into the pit. This exposes the top of the instrumentation rack on which the system controller and the magnetometer rest. Using the free black and orange lead connect the display battery (black to negative first). With the battery connected watch the display for three consecutive field readings, noting the second on which the battery light turns on and the field value. The three values should be consistent with 10y. The absolute value should be around 50,000y. The consistency is by far the more important of the two because occasionally elements of the display fail, making the numbers appear very different.

Comment: Whoopee! A+. A+. A+ !!!

5.   Although Professor Radcliffe-Brown's definition of political organization is to some extent correct, it is both inadequate and inaccurate, especially in its qualifications of the nebulous tenet; political organization is the component of social order, which serves to both stabilize and propagate the social order. To say that political organization is the force that unifies society is to say very little, indeed. The implication that this cohesion is efficacious only within a demarcated boundary under the auspices of a codified instrument of judicious authority is preposterous, when viewed in terms of societies whose social awareness is little more complex than the pectic bond between pack animals.

Comment: A prose that shoots itself in both feet. It has no feeling for the shape and rhythm of a single sentence, and this blindness blurs the focus and jumbles the sequence of the argument. Here is a perfect instance of what The Official Style, in its Social Science version, does to the quality of student thought. A style like this almost prohibits you from thinking through a problem clearly. No student writes like this naturally. He or she has to be taught this stylistic self-interference ritual. The literacy crisis, all this is to say, has been partly created by the academic versions of The Official Style, not imposed on higher education from the outside.

Let's start with the first sentence.   Sure, the semicolon after "tenet" and the comma after "order" are wrong, but these punctuation errors don't create the main problem - all that tentative, unfocussed, and self-contradictory action.   Radcliffe-Brown is both correct and inaccurate, but does the inaccuracy fall in the "nebulous tenet" or in its "qualifications"? Here, doing a PM routine as I have done really just serves to begin to tell us why The Official Style so often acts as a impenetrable barrier to clear thinking.   Look at all the potential actions swimming aimlessly about in this "sentence": define, organize, qualify, organize (again), serve, stabilize, propagate. No central action is being established from which the others can devolve. Back again to "Who's kicking Who?" **Prof. Radcliffe-Brown defines** . . . . To find out what he defines, you must consult the next sentence: **political organization is the force that unifies society.** Alas, according to this writer, this definition is both a definition and a part of that same definition, a qualification of a nebulous tenet. So murky is the prose that this writer makes a fundamental logical error without noticing it. But when we see that this has happened, we see that the first two sentences say the same thing. The correct/inadequate/inaccurate muddle means that the definition is *tautological.* The stabilize/propagate/unifies cluster means *preserves.* So we can revise: "Prof. Radcliffe-Brown defines political organization as the force which unifies society. But this definition is tautological! "

The last sentence has me upon thorns because I don't know what a "pectic bond between pack animals" means. But here's a try: "And not only tautological but preposterous: cohesion can work without a boundary or a codified instrument - look at the pectic bond between pack animals."

Revision: Prof. Radcliffe-Brown defines political organization as the force which unifies society. But this definition is tautological! And not only tautological, but preposterous: cohesion can work without a boundary or a codified instrument - look at the pectic bond between pack animals."

GRADUATE PROSE

The force of The Official Style operates if anything more strongly in graduate-student writing than in undergraduate prose. Graduate students are trainees for guild membership, and the best way to prove that you deserve membership is to write as the members write - and, if possible, more so. As a result, graduate-student writing at its worst often reads like a parody of the professional style in question. And it almost invariably sacrifices focus and power to a tedious series of unnecessary qualifications. It is often the hardest prose of all to revise. My revisions are beginning suggestions only.

1. A perfect example of the resultant polluted fragmentation of the Russian intelligentsia may be seen in the characters of Dostoevsky's The Idiot, who have a desperate awareness of the uncertain ground of their actions that causes them to hurl themselves towards a decisive event - revolution, crime, suicide, libertinism, religious extremism - in the hope that the external situation thus created will deprive them of choice and impose unity on their personalities.

Revision: The characters in Dostoevsky's The Idiot illustrate this polluted fragmentation of the Russian intelligentsia. Because they know they stand on uncertain ground, they hurl themselves towards a decisive event - revolution, crime, suicide, libertinism, religious extremism - hoping to find an external situation that will impose a single personality upon them.

2.   As a life-bringer and a death-dealer the old man contains his own opposites, and the hero's destruction of the dualistic greybeard provides a metaphor for the psychological process of incorporating the shadow, or dark side of the personality into the self for the purpose of achieving wholeness. The archetype of the Self represents the fusion of the various components of the psyche into a comprehensive entity, and this paradoxical union of opposites prefigures the phenomenon of rebirth and transfiguration.

Revision: Both life-bringer and death-dealer, the old man contains his own opposites.   The hero, by destroying him, symbolically incorporates the dark side of the personality into himself and thus makes himself whole. The archetypal self fuses the psyche's components into one, and this paradoxical union prefigures rebirth and transfiguration.

3. Behavior, words and body movements are gestures that evoke similar, identical and unique responses or reactions to the individual or community initiating the gesture. Paradoxically, gestures which create immediate perceptions, may direct or misdirect the person or community trying to interpret the motivation or meaning behind those gestures.

Revision: Behavior, words, and gestures evoke similar responses. But sometimes the gestures may be misinterpreted.

Comment: Does this somewhat deflationary translation leave anything out?

4. At this stage of the development of the spirit archetype, furthermore, the internalized Spirit would "miraculously" intervene to save the child from death, in spite of the unremitting perilousness of his adventures.

Revision: The internalized Spirit, when the spirit archetype has developed thus far, "miraculously" intervenes to preserve the child from his perils.

Comment: I guess.

5. Sex and violence: the two pursuits which express man's strongest physical urges. Every age must cope with them, must devise systems that allow release yet preserve a modicum of control. For the Elizabethans that control almost evaporated. The medieval church had ritualized sex and violence, defined their role in the cosmos. Expanding beyond these religious strictures, the Renaissance intellect faced emotional chaos. Therefore, a cultural preoccupation with these impulses evolved, which only our own age, emerging from the repressive safeguards of Puritanism and Victorianism, can match.

Comment: Hosannah!

PROFESSORIAL PROSE

No miraculous stylistic transformation occurs when a Ph.D. turns the graduate student caterpillar into a professorial butterfly. The following passages offer, naturally enough, the same formulaic Official Style tedium they inspire in the students who read them.

1.   At the center of any theory of a science of society is an image of man, a conception of him as a particular kind of creature, defined by his powers and liabilities.

Comment: The mixture as before:

At the center

of any theory

of a science

of society

is an image

of man . . .

Revision here exposes an embarrassing triviality of thought.

Revision: Any science of society presents, at its center, a particular conception of man.

2. Perception is the process of extracting information from stimulation emanating from the objects, places, and events in the world around us.

Revision: Perception extracts information from the world around us.

3. The notion of a process of abstraction at a perceptual level is not a new one.

Revision: Abstraction at a perceptual level is not a new idea.

4. An excellent example of use of the most economical distinctive feature for making a perceptual decision is an experiment by Yonas.

Revision: Yonas demonstrated, in an exemplary experiment, the most economical distinctive feature in a perceptual decision.

5. If we want to facilitate abstraction of a relation (and we often do in educational situations), we can draw attention to it by enhancing the feature contrast, or by providing uncluttered examples of the invariant property.

Comment: Look at the "shun" words:
> If we want to facilitate abstrac*tion* of a rela*tion* (and we often do in
> educa*tional* situa*tions*), we can draw atten*tion* . . .

Beyond this, I don't know what the passage means and so cannot revise it. If you know, give it a try.

6. The concept of role differentiation in any social system may be defined as the structures of distribution of the members of the system among the various positions and activities distinguished in the system, and hence the differential arrangement of the members of the system.

Comment: Unless I have missed an episode here, this is a classic tautology.   And Good Grief, Charlie Brown, look at the prepositions: The concept **of** role differentiation **in** any social system may be defined as the structures **of** distribution **of** the members **of** the system **among** various positions and activities distinguished **in** the system, and hence the differential arrangement **of** the members **of** the system.

Revision: Role differentiation means that different people play different roles.

7. We feel that a number of books on reading have failed in what should be an important function, that of providing the psychological and linguistic concepts that will give the student of reading insight into the learning process and what it is that must be learned to be a good reader.

Revision: Many books on reading do not provide the psychological and linguistic concepts needed to understand what a good reader must know. (LF. 59%)

8. The most eloquent testimony of the flexibility and the durability of the academy as an institution is that offered by Arcadia, the pan-Italian federation of local academies founded in Rome in 1690 by the former members of the salon of Queen Christina of Sweden for the purpose of reforming Italian literature in accordance with the literary models of the High Renaissance.

Comment: Laundry-list historical prose which tries to put too much in one sentence. If you break it into two sentences, you can almost live with the prepositional phrases.

Revisions:

1. Arcadia offers the most eloquent testimony of the flexibility and durability of the academy as an institution. This pan-Italian federation of local academies was founded in Rome in 1690 by the former members of the salon of Queen Christina of Sweden, who wanted to reform Italian literature according to High Renaissance models.

2. Arcadia, perhaps, testifies most eloquently to the flexible durability of the academy as an institution. This pan-Italian federation of local academies, founded in Rome in 1690 by former courtiers of Queen Christina of Sweden, aimed to reform Italian literature according to High Renaissance models.

9. In this paper, we replace the realistic radiative transfer process by an escape probability method for a slab geometry (of infinite area but finite thickness). We make this approximation in order to be able to explore a wide range of parameter space.   Modifications would have to be made to the escape probability-optical depth relation for a spherical geometry.

Comment: Pretty good stuff. Let it be.

10. An awareness of the role of the recording industry in the dissemination of folk music and musical styles is not new; to date, however, there has been little consideration of the importance of commercial recording in relation to Irish folk music.

Comment: A straight PM repair: An awareness **of** the role **of** the recording industry **in** the dissemination **of** folk music and musical styles **is** not new; to date, however, **there has been** little consideration **of** the importance **of** commercial recording **in** relation **to** Irish folk music.

Revision: We have always known that the recording industry disseminated folk music and musical styles; to date, however, we have not considered how it influenced Irish folk music.

11. From this description, it can be seen that a positive incremental voltage applied to a device biased beyond the peak in the velocity-field curve causes a decrease in the terminal current due to the formation of the dipole layer. This is a negative resistance.

Comment: Needs only applause.

12. The lot of the prisoner on the battlefield of the gunpowder age benefited from the generalization of the principle of ransom.

Comment: Standard problem. Easy fix.

Revision: When, in the gunpowder age, the principle of ransom was generalized, the lot of the battlefield prisoner improved.

13. What makes episodes of this sort so difficult for the modern reader to visualize, if visualized to believe in, if believed in to understand, is precisely their nakedly face-to-face quality, their offering and delivery of death over distances at which suburbanites swap neighbourly gardening hints, their letting of blood and infliction of pain in circumstances of human congestion we expect to experience only at cocktail parties or tennis tournaments.

Comment: Another long sentence, but this time the writer has tried to control it, shape it, give it some climactic focus. Contrast it with the shapeless jumbos we've dissected above. Pretty hard to improve this prose without rewriting it completely, but I'll try. Have I made it better or worse?

Revision: What makes such episodes so difficult for the modern reader to visualize, if visualized to believe in, if believed in to understand, is precisely their nakedly face-to-face quality. They offer and deliver death over distances at which suburbanites swap neighbourly gardening hints, let blood and inflict pain in crowds we experience only at cocktail parties or tennis tournaments.

14. The same scheme was adopted for the promotion of the study of the church fathers and of the implications of humanism for ecclesiastical reform by the Tridentine enthusiasts in the entourage of the young cardinal Carlo Borromeo during the pontificate of his uncle, Pius IV.

Comment: Same old problems:
The same scheme

    was adopted

    for the promotion

    of the study

    of the church fathers and

    of the implications

    of humanism

    for ecclesiastical reform

    by the Tridentine enthusiasts

    of the young cardinal Carlo Borromeo

    during the pontificate

    of his uncle, Pius IV.

You get hopelessly lost trying to remember what goes with, or affects, what. A sentence like this really does resemble a sausage, stuffed with prepositional phrases. To figure out what is going on, you need to outline the sentence:

The Tridentine enthusiasts adopted the same scheme
   1) to promote study of the church fathers
   2) to promote study of the implications of humanism
With this outline in mind, here's a tentative revision. I wouldn't give it more than a C+. Improve on it.

Revision: During Pius IV's pontificate, Tridentine enthusiasts in the entourage of his young nephew, cardinal Carlo Borromeo, adopted the same scheme. They used it to promote study of the church fathers and of humanism's implications for ecclesiastical reform.

15. On the other hand, the firmness (or rigidity) of some university faculties, including my own, in resisting the awarding of credit for remedial work arises directly out of their sense of vulnerability of the standards for college level work, standards already weakened by diversity, competition, a shocking grade inflation since the mid-1960s, the powerful pressure of the market for enrollments and the call for "relevance." The fact that there are differences on this matter, both of views and of practice, is the best evidence for how soft is the concept of academic standards in higher education, and consequently how vulnerable those standards are to market pressures, especially the pressure to maintain enrollment at all costs.

Comment: Archetypal absent-minded Official Style, Social Science Version.

Revision: Some college faculties have resisted giving credit for remedial work so firmly because they fear that college-level standards, already weakened by grade inflation, "relevance," and enrollment competition, will collapse. The widely different views about remedial credit themselves show how fragile university standards remain, and how vulnerable to market and enrollment pressures.

16. During the year ahead it is my intention to engage a larger number of incumbent faculty in the governance process.

Comment: The President of the Academic Senate delivered himself of this unintentional Official Style self-parody.

Revision: During the coming year, I shall ask more faculty members to participate in Senate business.

17. The limitations along another dimension of sociobiological explanations of human social activity can be illustrated by considering the Cartesian product of the act/action distinction with the distinction between activities which have a biological origin in an inherited genetic program selected by Darwinian processes, and those which have their origin in the creative cognitive activities of men as conscious social beings.

Comment: Sorry, I just can't understand this, and so cannot revise it. Give it a try if you know what it means.

18. The progress of the discipline of psychoanalysis is expressed perhaps most obviously in its theory of transference and the therapeutic effects of the interpretation of transference.

Comment: An old favorite of mine because blurring of natural subject and verb is so total and uniform. You have to choose what to stress yourself.

Revisions:
1.   Psychoanalysis has progressed most obviously in the theory of transference and its therapeutic effects.
2.   The theory of transference, and the therapeutic effects of its interpretation, perhaps express best the progress of psychoanalysis.
3.   The progress of psychoanalysis as a discipline is perhaps best seen in transference and its interpretation.

19. My main reason for writing this book is to reassert the methodological priority of the search for the laws of history in the science of man. There is an urgency associated with this rededication, which grows in direct proportion to the increase in the funding and planning of anthropological research and especially to the role anthropologists have been asked to assume in the planning and carrying out of international development programs. A general theory of history is required if the expansion of disposable research funds is to result in something other than the rapid growth in the amount of trivia being published in the learned journals.

Comment: Much academic writing is less bad than - like this passage - simply thoughtless and formulaic. The "The fact of the matter in a case of this sort is such as to require a blah, blah, blah" kind of sentence comes naturally to someone for whom prose is not a self-consciously felt means of expression. If it goes on twice as long as it needs to, well, just skip most of it, as most people do. Students find themselves in a particularly virulent form of this downward spiral. Their papers are read by people who write this way and expect this kind of prose. Why not just go with the flow?

Revision: I wrote this book to argue that we must continue to seek the laws of history.   The more carefully planned and widely funded anthropological research becomes, the more we need a general theory of history.   This need becomes especially pronounced when anthropologists are asked to create international development programs.

20. Our lives and the world we are part of are uniquely multifaceted and a sense of identity with this pluralism is expressed in musical terms. The fact that there are today so many varied aesthetic attitudes shaping the musical structures and that these approaches to creativity are seemingly disparate is consciously understood and challenged. That as we live side by side and with and among so many attitudes, so music's language is a host that embraces a wide range of possibilities.

Comment: Art criticism seems to invite this kind of pretentious guff, for some reason. Any revision becomes ironic deflation.

Revision: Musical aesthetics today is as pluralistic as the other arts and the society which supports them.